The Lazy Girl's

EASY

Weight Loss Method

**The Secret to Losing the Fat *Without* Exercise
or Giving Up the Bacon, Burgers, and Burritos**

By Sment Bronzini

CONTENTS

You're a Lazy Girl

The first step is admitting you have a problem. Like I was not so long ago, you're overweight. No, it's not because you're big-boned, or just because you're getting older and "that's what happens." No. You have fat, probably around your thighs, butt, belly, and maybe in your back, your chest or even your cankles, er, ankles. Bottom line – you have some weight to lose. Maybe it's 200 pounds, maybe it's 15. But you don't know where else to turn.

You know that typical diets aren't for you. You don't want to go without carbs. Carbs are freaking delicious. You don't want to sit there and boil flavorless skinless chunks of chicken. You don't particularly like the idea of eating eggs without the yolks. You don't want unflavored yogurt to be your breakfast. You wince at the words "multi-grain," "gluten-free," "skim," and worst of all, "low-fat." And when a dish is made with a low-calorie substitute, you can't believe it's not *better*.

But besides the unappealing diets that are either too difficult, too expensive, too hard to maintain, or just plain unappealing, you also know there are lots of gimmicks out there that aren't going to work either. You know there is no magic pill that will "burn fat." Not that you haven't tried your fair share of miracle products. You know that any of those infomercial gadgets you buy that promise toned, sleek abs and cellulite-free thighs will either not give you what it promises, or will gather dust after you use it once.

Perhaps more important though, is one major fact: you are inherently – let's face it – lazy. You are not going to get up at four in the morning before work and jog for ten miles. It's cold out! You know that if you chopped up tuna and celery (hold the mayo, of course) and prepared it for lunch every day, you wouldn't end up taking it to work. You've thought about doing squats, leg lifts, and hitting the gym, but hey, you're tired at the end of a long day. Besides, you've found that those exercises don't make the fat go away. Your gym membership card, if it exists, has gone unused for quite some time. You'd cancel the membership, but you tell yourself that maybe someday you'll miraculously have the energy to start going again.

Besides, you love food. Who doesn't? You look forward to meals. They're a bright spot in your day. And you're not particularly picky, as long as it tastes good. You love cheeseburgers, ice cream, French fries, pizza, quesadillas, spaghetti, steak, baked potatoes, eggs, hashed browns, waffles… need I go on?

You've come to the right place. This book is designed for the Lazy Girl who wants to lose weight. This diet plan (if you can really call it that) is simple, and that's perfect for Lazy Girls. Even the book itself is short, because what Lazy Girl wants to sit reading a 250-page diet book before even having a clue what the diet involves?

But even though this diet plan is easy, that doesn't mean it requires no effort from you. For it to work, you have to follow it to a T. You have to commit to it and its rules. If you do that, you'll be surprised how well it works and just how simple it is.

So who am I? I'm not a doctor, a nutritionist, or a dietician. In fact, I have no certification in the medical or health fields whatsoever. I am simply a Lazy Guy (yes, the original book was for men) who has stumbled upon something amazing. I love food, and yet I found that it didn't love me back. Realizing I was not happy with my body, I tried all kinds of things to lose weight, but none were effective or long-lasting. I read about something called "calorie counting," and started to wonder – if all that matters is that you take in fewer calories than you burn, why not make those calories something you'll enjoy?

It seemed too good to be true. So I put it to the test. I followed the exact methods outlined in this guide, and to my pleasant surprise, it worked. People couldn't believe I had lost so much weight when they heard I never gave up the foods I loved.
And if it worked for me, I know it can work for you.

How It Works

So what is "calorie counting" anyway? Sounds not only complicated and a pain in the ass, but kind of nerdy, right? Well, it usually is. And people think that if you're counting calories, that basically means you can only eat rice cakes and Lean Cuisines®.

But here comes the nice thing about being a fat (or slightly chunky) chick who wants to lose weight: You can "count calories" without limiting yourself to typical "diet" foods.

Unfortunately for you, men's metabolisms make it easier for them to lose weight than women. At least that's my understanding. Whatever the reason, men need more calories than women do, even if they're the same age, height, and weight. That's why the original book was specifically geared for guys. But the truth is, it works for women just as well.

You really can eat hamburgers, ice cream, pizza, hot dogs, chips, fries, etc. and still lose weight. And I don't mean low-calorie or fat-free versions of the above either. I'm talking about the above dishes from your favorite fast food restaurants, not from the healthy section at your local supermarket.

Here's why it works. Basically, your body is a machine. Even if your particular machine is adorned with bra strap fallout and thunder thighs. It's still a machine. It requires fuel to make it work. That's what food is for. And that doesn't just mean energy so you can go run a marathon. Your body needs fuel even if you just sit around all day and watch soap operas.

Yes, your body burns the energy you get from food on its own, just in carrying out its own daily processes – keeping your heart beating, your blood warm, your lungs breathing, and probably a whole lot of things I don't even know about.

But imagine you're filling up your car with gasoline. You need to do that so it can function, so it can take you places. But what happens if you overfill it? Well, in the case of this less-than-ideal analogy, the gasoline may leak out the side of the tank and end up on your shoes.

But if you do the same thing with your body, that is, take in more fuel than it needs just to function, that fuel doesn't just spill out your mouth (unless you're a supermodel with a strong gag reflex.) No, it ends up being stored on your body as – you guessed it – fat.

The alternative, however, is the key to this diet. It's actually pretty simple, and no scientist or nutritionist will deny this: *If you take in fewer calories than your body uses, your body uses your own fat for its missing energy.*

Pretty cool, right? I guess if we take this further, we could just fast for a week and lose a ton of weight, right?

Nope, sorry. It doesn't work that way. You really can't safely lose more than a pound of fat per week. Try anything more severe and you're bound to start losing muscle and find yourself malnourished. In fact, if you did that, you'd find that your metabolism compensates by slowing down, and your body actually becomes *less* efficient at burning its own fat. Not only would that be unhealthy, but you wouldn't be able to keep it up for very long.

But the fact remains that if you can manage your food intake just right, you can make your body rely on your own stored fat, use it for energy, and decrease your weight.

One pound a week might seem slow. But realize this: in just three months, you will have lost *over* 10 pounds. Better yet, unlike pretty much every other diet out there, this one doesn't make you live in misery. You'll see why as we move on.

So what's next? Now, we need to find out how many calories you can take in each day to lose that pound of fat per week.

There are a lot of calorie-consumption calculators on the web, but below you'll find a list of my favorites, which were up and running as of press time. It's also included in the Appendix for easy reference.

Basically, scientists and nutritionists have determined that each pound of fat we have equates to about 3,500 calories. Let's assume you're currently not gaining any weight, but are not losing any either. If you reduce the amount of calories you take in each week by 3,500, you will lose a pound of fat. Conveniently, 3,500 divides by 7 (the number of days in a week), equaling 500. So each day, if you consume 500 fewer calories than you normally do, you will lose that pound of fat in a week. Don't worry, the online calculators figure this out for you.

In other words, for every 3,500 calories you *don't* eat each week (compared to the number it takes to stay at your current weight), you will lose a pound. And the way that makes the most sense to decrease your calorie intake, is to do it on a daily basis, by taking in 500 fewer calories each day.

Pay attention to each calculator's specific information. Some of them are set up to tell you how many calories you need to take in to *maintain* your weight. That's not what you want. So for those calculators, subtract 500, and you'll get the number of calories to take in to *lose* weight.

Again, now that you know the specifics, there's always the temptation – why not cut 7,000 calories and lose two pounds every week? Again, you could, but most dieticians agree that's not only unhealthy, but it's really hard to do. You'll end up feeling hungry and possibly weak. And then you won't want to continue on this plan at all.

So you may be wondering, isn't this just calorie counting? It's cool and all, but what makes this diet special again?

The answer is that, like any diet, calorie counting only works as long as you're willing to do it. Most calorie counters restrict themselves to low-calorie, low-fat (a.k.a. flavorless) items in order to not go over their limit. Why? Most dieters, like you, are women! And women typically don't have as large a calorie allowance as men do. So they think you have to look for the items with the fewest calories, and therefore, taste.

I'm going to show you that you can still eat your favorite foods on this plan, as long as you're smart and careful.

Get started by using one of the calorie-consumption calculators below. If you're confused, or need more guidance, you can come back to this part later. But this is the time to get excited. You're on your way to a thinner you, all without giving up the joy of food! Remember, some of them show the number of daily calories you'll have to eat to *maintain* your current weight. Subtract 500, and you have the magic number, the amount of calories you can eat each day to lose a pound of fat per week.

A Few Reliable Calorie-Consumption Calculators
http://www.mayoclinic.com/health/calorie-calculator/NU00598
http://www.freedieting.com/tools/calorie_calculator.htm
http://calorieneedscalculator.com/
http://www.healthyweightforum.org/eng/calculators/calories-required/
http://www.caloriesperhour.com/
http://www.hpathy.com/healthtools/calories-need.asp

How to Do It

So let's get down to the nitty gritty. I'm going to use Britney as an example. Britney is 35 years old, 5 feet, 4 inches, and 150 pounds. Chances are you are a different age, height and weight. Don't worry about that. This works regardless of whether you're a short, old, extremely fat Lazy Girl, or a tall, young, semi-fat Lazy Girl. In fact, I've purposely chosen a woman that's not really that heavy at all, to show you that losing weight by eating "non-diet" foods is possible even when your daily allowance for calories is low.

Britney goes to one of the online calorie-consumption calculators. She enters all her info, but it asks her how "active" she is. My personal recommendation is that unless you run a marathon everyday (due to the title of this book, you probably don't), you should mark yourself as "couch potato." Most of the calculators euphemistically call that "sedentary." (There are several reasons I recommend this, even though you may actually *be* more active. See the section later titled Exercise. And no, don't worry, as mentioned before, exercise is not required.)

Next, the calculator spits out Britney's results. It tells her that she can consume about 1,200 calories per day to lose a pound each week. On her particular calculator, she rounded down from 1,223. If you want to be more exact, you can, but make sure you don't round *up*.

As I alluded to, chances are that your number is higher, meaning you can take in *more* calories each day. In fact, the great thing is that the fatter you currently are, the easier this will be to start off!

Britney's mission? All she needs to do each day is make sure that she eats no more than the total calories she's allowed: 1,200. But as long as she keeps it under than number, the sky's the limit! She can eat *anytime* during the day. She can eat *whatever* she wants. If she chooses to eat only sticks of butter (810 calories each), she can. If she wants only pancakes (170 calories each at Denny's®, not counting extra butter or syrup), she can.

The only thing you need to watch out for is quantity. That's the "catch," I guess you could say. But you'll get used to it. When you see that you're actually losing weight without breaking a sweat, *and* still getting to eat your favorite foods, you'll see that quantity is less and less important. You'll soon come to realize that this is like no diet you ever knew existed.

The Numbers

So how do we find out how many calories are in everything? As you may or may not know, largely because of government regulations, most packaged food at the supermarket has a big label on it that tells you how many calories are in it.

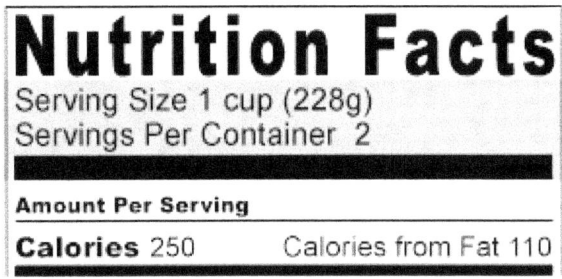

That makes it easy to count when you're buying something at said supermarket. But, Lazy Girls don't necessarily get their food primarily from supermarkets. What about when you're going to a fast food restaurant? Actually, most of the major fast food restaurant chains either have the information available in the restaurant, or on their website. There are also a myriad of books which you can buy online or through your local bookstore which are full of the same information. The only problem with a book containing nutritional information is that it can go out of date. New items won't be in the book, and items that are no longer sold will remain in print. Thus, you won't find listings for those books here. But they're easy to find, if you choose to. (Including them here would also make this book very thick, which would deter Lazy Girls from buying it.) Other resources I've found especially convenient are various applications on your iPhone® or other similar device. Many of these programs are free, as well. They often have a ton of well-known establishments with the calorie count of all their dishes listed. Many of these apps even let you enter the food and it will keep track of the exactly total of calories. So while you're sitting on the subway, in the bus, or (parked) in your car, you can easily plan out your breakfast, lunch, or dinner.

As you can see, there are a lot of Nutritional Information Sources (I'll call them N.I.S.) from which to choose. You can also find quite a few listed in the Appendix of this book. Later, we'll tackle the problem of eating in restaurants or people's homes, where clearly, the caloric content of every item is not exactly readily available.

A Sample Day

So since I promised that you could eat those foods you love, we'll do an example that way.

Let's go back to Britney. She is driving to work. Usually, she would grab a breakfast sandwich at a drive-thru on her way. And guess what? Her new diet doesn't put a stop to that. So she goes to McDonald's®. She refers to any one of the Nutritional Information Sources (N.I.S.) mentioned above (or did it online the night before), and realized that there are a lot of choices!

Decisions, decisions! She still can't believe that her new "diet" allows her to order a regular breakfast item at a fast food drive-thru. She knows she only has 1,200 calories for the day, so she automatically nixes some higher-calorie meals right off the bat. She's not going to get something that's 600 calories, because then her lunch and dinner won't be very satisfying. (Although if a big breakfast is more important to you than a big dinner, go for it!) So she opts for the Egg McMuffin® for only 300 calories! The clerk says, "Do you want the meal?" She hadn't thought of this. She checks her facts and sees that the "hash brown" is 150 calories. It's doable, but she decides she can do without it this time. In so doing, she saves that 150 calories for later in the day.

She takes out a little scrap of paper and a pen and quickly jots down:

> Monday, March 3
> Egg McMuffin®   300

If that works best for you, by all means, do so. But in the Appendix you'll find a Calorie Tracker sheet which you may wish to use. Again, there are plenty of smartphone apps as well as websites that allow you to track calories each day.

Okay, let's see if you're keeping track. How many calories does Britney have left for the day?

We take her total allowance of 1,200 and subtract the 300 for breakfast. She has 900 left.

Britney gets to work, feeling good. But suddenly, an obstacle in her path – one of her co-workers has brought donuts! They look tasty, and she wants one. Can she have it? Yes! She can have it and still lose weight today! Of course, that means she has fewer calories left in the day for later. So she takes the donut and sets it on her desk. After all, she's not sure if she's going to eat it, and she's not exactly going to say, "Wait, let me check how many calories this has first." Then, she discreetly peeks at her N.I.S., in this case, a book she picked up at Barnes and Noble®. She's not sure where the donut's from, but she's found out that a Winchell's® Old Fashioned Glazed Donut is a whopping 410 calories. And she knows this particular pastry is the same size and description as the Winchell's® one. If Britney eats it, *which she could*, she'd have about 500 calories left for the day. Again, it's doable, but she doesn't want to be hungry later, so she skips it. If you were in Britney's place, and you can't muster up the will power, don't feel bad. Next time you'll be stronger. Or, eat half (for 205) calories, and throw the other half out before your mouth gets a hold of it! The best solution would have just been to say, "No thanks," when offered. But again, whether to eat it or not is a choice you make, and either way, you can still lose the weight. Pretty cool, right?

This time though, Britney was able to pass on it, and you'll see how nice that will work out later.

Lunch time! The girls from work want to go out for lunch. Oh no, Britney's first day on this new diet and she's being tested again already! Wait a second, she can do this. Her buddies say they're going to Sharky's®, a Mexican chain restaurant. If you don't have them in your area, they're similar to La Salsa®, Baja Fresh®, Chipotle®, and Poquito Mas®. She quickly checks her N.I.S. and sees that some menu items would take up her entire day's allowance. "But I thought we could eat our favorite foods on this diet!" you scream. Hold on now. If Britney really wanted to, she could order one of the high-calorie items, eat half now and maybe have the rest for dinner. Hey, it's still a diet, right?

But she doesn't want anyone to know she's doing anything out of the ordinary. She remembers that after her 300-calorie breakfast, she has 900 left. Sharky's® Oven Baked Chicken Burrito is 1,310 calories. Too much. She discovers their Santa Fe Chicken Burrito is 720 calories. Doable, but that would make dinner really tough. What about tacos? How could anyone eat tacos and lose weight? But she can! Sharky's® Chicken Gringo Taco is only 140 calories! She decides to get two of them, for a 280 calorie total. She could have them, and still have 620 calories for dinner. What about chips though? They don't even list them on their nutritional info! She could either skip them, or look for tortilla chips from another N.I.S. But that would really cut into the calories left for dinner. So she decides to skip the chips, and enjoy the tacos a la carte.

She adds to her list:

Monday, March 3	
Egg McMuffin®	300
Two Chicken Gringo Tacos	280
TOTAL SO FAR	580

She gets home and is feeling great with her success. Dinner has a lot of options in store, but Britney has to remember not to go over her remaining 620 calories. Could she manage a hamburger? She checks her N.I.S. and finds out that most of the fast food chains offer some kind of burger for 620 or fewer calories. She decides to go with Wendy's® and their best option. To her shock, she sees that their quarter-pound single burger is only 470 calories! That would leave her with 150 calories. Should she get the Value size fries (210 calories) and only have half? How about the Junior Vanilla Frosty™ (150 calories)? She goes for the sweet option, and passes on the fries this time.

She adds to her list:

Monday, March 3

Egg McMuffin®	300
Two Chicken Gringo Tacos	280
Hamburger	470
Frosty™	150
TOTAL	1,200

Today's been the first day of Britney's new "diet," and she was able to eat at McDonald's®, Sharky's®, and Wendy's® without having some meal with a little heart icon next to it or a tiny bowl of salad leaves with no dressing. She had eggs, tacos, a burger, and a shake! She can't believe that she's going to lose weight this way!

By the way, you may notice that she ended up with exactly 1,200 calories in this example. It won't always work that way. This isn't an exact science. The online calorie-consumption calculators are dishing out your data based on the average woman of that height, weight, and age. Everybody's metabolism varies slightly, so 10 calories here or there is not going to make a big difference. I find it's better to err on the side of caution, and stay under your limit rather than go over.

More Sample Days

Britney can use her 1,200 calories in an infinite number of ways. Here's a few to give you an idea of just how liberating this diet really is:

Item	Calories
Pop Tart® (Brown Sugar Cinnamon)	210
Arby's Melt®	302
Jalapeno Bites from Arby's®	305
BURGER KING® WHOPPER JR.® with Cheese	380
Total	1,197

Item	Calories
Krispy Kreme® Chocolate Iced Glazed donut	250
Macaroni Grill® Grilled Chicken Spiedini	410
El Pollo Loco® BRC Burrito	430
El Pollo Loco® Mashed Potatoes	110
Total	1,200

Item	Calories
Starbucks® Iced Hazelnut Hot Choc. (2% milk)	350
Subway® Buffalo Chicken 6" sandwich	420
Taco Bell® Nachos Supreme	430
Total	1,200

Item	Calories
Noah's® Everything Bagel Thin Single	160
Noah's® Onion and Chive Cream Cheese Shmear	120
Carl's Jr.® Buttermilk Ranch Chkn. Tender ™ Wrapper	290
Carl's Jr.® Kids Fries	240
KFC® Tender Roast Sandwich	380
Total	1,190

Item	Calories
Multi-Grain Cheerios® (cup, dry)	110
Jack in the Box® Chicken Fajita Pita®	280
Chili's® Classic Sirloin	250
Chili's® Sweet Corn on the Cob with Butter	220
Chili's® Applewood Smoked Bacon (3 strips)	90
Chili's® Spicy Garlic and Lime Shrimp (6 pcs.)	130
Bud Light® (12-oz. can)	110
Total	1,190

Dining Out

It really is pretty simple. However, the most difficult part about the diet, in my opinion, is counting calories for food that doesn't come with a label. What happens when you're at a restaurant or at someone's house? It can be tough to judge.

The first thing to do is to prepare in advance. I'm not going to advocate starving yourself all day in preparation for a dinner out, but I do think you should alter your meals based on what you're doing later. For instance, if Britney is allowing herself 1,200 calories a day, it makes more sense for her to eat a smaller breakfast and smaller lunch than usual if she knows she's going to possibly eat a lot that night. Fasting isn't a good idea for many reasons, but eating very small portions can at least help you get by. In fact, on the last sample day in the previous section, you saw that Britney had a relatively low calorie count for breakfast and lunch so that he could have a lot of flexibility at dinner.

So shifting your allotment of calories around based on your plans for the day is a good trick. In the previous case, when dinner comes along, Britney will have a decent amount of calories to work with. But that doesn't mean she can eat anything she wants. The longer you've been doing this, the better you will get at "eyeing" the calories. In other words, if you see that a grilled chicken dish is being served, you might be able to guess its calorie content because you've eaten a similar dish before that had a label. If you have a choice, definitely try and go for the smaller portions. You can also save a lot of calories by not getting an appetizer, opting out of dessert, or getting rice instead of fries.

But for some people, the best choice is to order all of the above, and just not eat the whole thing. That can not only save on embarrassment from your girlfriends ("What, you're on a diet?"), but can also allow you to feel less limited. In other words, this way you may not feel like you're on a diet. A bite of chocolate cake won't fill you up, but at least you'll have a delicious mouthful (instead of a highly-caloric slice) and still know that you're losing weight.

After the meal, use a N.I.S. listed in this book (or one you find on your own) to figure out roughly how many calories you ate. If you overate, you'll know for next time. If you ate less than your limit, you can have a snack when you get home. That probably won't be the case though.

Again, eating out is definitely doable on this diet, but not as easy as being your normal lazy self and getting fast food. However, if you have any choice in the selection of the venue, try going for a big chain restaurant. They often have their nutritional information listed on their webpage.

You will also find yourself doing a lot of guesstimating. Just because you've seen an apple listed for, say, 100 calories, doesn't mean that every apple will be that. If you find a particularly large apple, you've got to assume it's more, maybe 140 or 150. It's not an exact science, but estimating on the cautious side (meaning counting it as more calories rather than less) will help you in the long run.

Writing down a number that's not really accurate doesn't hurt anybody but yourself.

Salads

As I mentioned, if you think your entrée might be heavy in calories, try and cut some other calories by swapping the butter-drenched baked potato for a rice pilaf or side salad. But at the same time, beware of things that seem low in calories that aren't. A lot of salads have tons of cheese, olives, or things like prosciutto, which can quickly make them just as high in calories as a dish you'd prefer, like onion rings. And that's not even counting the dressing. So if you're into salads, great, but go light on the dressing. And as with anything, check the calories. Getting it without dressing works, but it's kind of a miserable experience, from a Lazy Guy's perspective. Try putting on a tablespoon or two, mush it around, and that way you'll still enjoy the flavor.

Alcohol

Don't forget when you go out (or even at home), that you need to count *everything*. And that includes alcohol, as you saw in the More Sample Days section. And if you don't drink? Great. But if you do, be prepared to reconsider how often you're drinking and what you're drinking.

Most 12-ounce cans of beer are about 150 calories. And that's just *one*. Not only do most of us not stop there, but even if you drink one beer, that means eating less actual food to stay under your calorie limit. A four-ounce glass of most wines is roughly 100 calories. A vodka cran or gin and tonic is roughly 200 calories. Margaritas, piña coladas – they can go up into several hundred calories. Stay away from the fruity drinks, too, ladies. And since alcohol lowers your inhibitions, you're less likely to stick to your calorie limits while you're drinking anyway. So be careful.

Don't forget, some of the "light" beers are a little better for you, calorie-wise. But there are some truly low-calorie beers (under 100 calories) that you might want to consider, too. If you get teases from your cosmo-sipping girlfriends, tell them that *Sex and the City* came and went a long time ago. That may shut them up for a little while.

Soda, Tea, and Coffee

Alcohol is not the only type of drink that you have to consider when staying under your calorie limit. If you drink regular soda, check out the labels. They have a lot of calories. I happen to have grown up on diet soda, so I can drink it to my heart's content without adding any calories to my day. But for those of us that like the sugary stuff, think about it. Is that soda really worth it to you?

The nice thing is that there are quite a few sodas on the market now which have zero or almost zero calories, but taste a lot like their high-calorie equivalents. I'm a big fan of Pepsi One® and Coca-Cola Zero®. They both use different sweeteners than the normal diet cola drinks, and therefore manage to taste more like a regular soda. Even the energy drinks, ranging from Rockstar® to Powerade®, now offer low-calorie versions.

A *benefit* to diet sodas is that they can fill you up, at least temporarily, making you less hungry. So they're good in that regard too. When you drink them with a meal, they can make the meal feel more satisfying as well.

If you can't stomach the sugar-free sodas, go ahead and have your regular ones, but you may soon realize it's not worth it. Or, have half a can, pour it on ice, and you can get away with drinking less of it.

If you drink coffee or tea, some people say the caffeine is actually good for dieters because it speeds up your metabolism. But little good that's going to do if you're dumping sugar into that coffee or tea. Try one of the sugar substitutes. Experiment and figure out if you prefer the yellow, the blue, or the pink. Any of them will cut a lot of calories from your day – calories that you would otherwise have to track. When some know-it-all tries to tell you that you shouldn't be putting those "chemicals" into your body, first tell them you're not exactly a lab rat consuming your body weight worth of artificial sweeteners. Then tell them that if those "chemicals" help you lose weight, then your health will be improving anyway. If that still doesn't work, you can probably figure out what to tell them.

Water

And finally, in our beverage category, we need to deal with the big guy. If you're truly a Lazy Girl, you probably don't like drinking water. However, you've probably heard how drinking water is important not only in life in general, but a key factor in losing weight. I'm not sure how true this is, but I do know this: it helps to keep you full. I'm not saying a glass of water will stave off your craving for a slice of pizza, but I do know that when I'm super hungry, it's often because I'm dehydrated.

So if you can, try and drink water during the day. It'll make everything much easier.

Snacks

So far, we've mainly talked about breakfast, lunch, and dinner. On this eating plan, you get to eat the foods you've always liked. That may not leave tons of extra calories for little snacks in between.

However, with time, you will learn how to get the smaller burger, or skip the cheese this time, to save you calories for later in the day.

There's nothing wrong with having junk food around either. You'll quickly find that it doesn't fill you up too well, but sometimes just knowing that you're having it makes you feel more able to conquer this diet. Sometimes having half a snickers bar (half a two-ounce bar is 133 calories) makes everything a little easier.

But there are also some great options at supermarkets nowadays. You've no doubt seen various companies coming up with these "100-calorie packs." They're actually pretty good. They give you the flavor you crave, and they're pre-packaged to prevent you from going back to the bag after your hundred calories is "up."

Sugarless chewing gum is a great between-meals "snack" because it's virtually calorie-free (not zero calories though), it gives you a nice flavor, and it gives your mouth something to do besides eating.

But I Want Fries With That

Now even though this diet is for Lazy Girls, that doesn't mean that everything is a cinch. As you may have noticed, I've mentioned certain fast food items a la carte, or without things like French fries. But they're the best part, right?

Again, it's a numbers game. I've gotten used to skipping the fries, but sometimes I have them, too. Some of the sample days in the earlier section included them. However, *not* skipping that extra side dish might mean those calories come out of a later meal. Be careful not to give in to your "present" self if it means screwing your "future" self. You know what I mean? You don't want to insist on having those fries now and then leave yourself with 200 calories for dinner.

Another option, instead of foregoing the fries (or other delicious side dish) is to opt for the smaller "entre," such as a smaller burger, and then it will help the numbers work out.

But what I've found is that I really don't need *all* those fries. At McDonalds®, the small fries have 230 calories. If there's room for that in my day's calculations, I'll do it. But sometimes I'll take the fries out, lay 'em on a napkin, and divide them into two piles as carefully as I can. Can you guess the next part? I throw out one pile. How many calories am I left with? 115. It's like one of those 100-calorie packs but with fresh, hot, salty French fries! And if you really throw the other half in the trash *first*, you won't miss it. Add that to a Quarter Pounder® for 410 calories, and you've just eaten a burger and fries for 525 calories! It wasn't "light" or "lo-cal" or a "healthy" option either. Jared, eat your heart out!

Errors in Labels

While nutrition labels can really come in handy, there are some cases where they are not correct! I won't mention it by name, but one of the fast food restaurants has a chicken nachos dish that I used to regularly order. It was listed on their website at about 1,000 calories, so in the later stages of my diet, I really had to limit myself to during the day in order to feast on that delicacy at night. Problem was, I started noticing that the nachos were sometimes different. Some days there was more cheese, some days there were more chips, some days tomatoes were on top, some days they weren't there at all. I used to excitedly wait to see if it was going to be a heavy container. That would mean there was more in it that day, and I could still count it as 1,000 calories *because the website said so*. Of course, I was only hurting myself. I have since stopped eating their nachos. Anytime there's that much flexibility in how a dish is served, you know that you can't count on the N.I.S. for it.

There's even a website that claims to have nutritional information for all sorts of foods at a huge variety of restaurants. As I discovered, the information on the website is in large part updated by the site's users. I saw a lot of wrong information, or things that were just too good to be true. I've tried to list only websites and information sources in the Appendix that are reliable, but be careful if you venture out into other sources.

Quantity

As I said, you really can eat anything you like on this diet, as long as it falls into your calorie limit for the day. A small Dominos® pizza is about 1,200 calories. So technically, someone like Britney could eat an entire pizza each day of the week and still lose weight. But, will you want to? I mean, I *love* pizza, and I have done the above experiment, just to see if it would really work. But that means you get about two slices for breakfast, two for lunch, and then another two for dinner, and very little (or nothing) else! You might get kind of bored of that. But it shows the point that it's really not what you eat, but how much of it you eat.

Get in the habit of trying to eat just half of some of those delicious foods. I've had a half serving of nachos for 1,000 calories from a different restaurant (yes, I love nachos) once for dinner when I hadn't eaten too much that day for breakfast and lunch. It worked out great. But I find that you should cut the portion you're going to eat first, and toss (or store out of your sight) the rest of it. Otherwise, you'll be too tempted to just have that proverbial "one more bite," which ends up being fifteen more.

However, when you stop eating, give yourself ten minutes and you may notice that you feel full anyway.

So what if you're still hungry after eating? This might happen as you begin this eating plan, perhaps because you're just not used to it. Your stomach is an expandable organ, and if you usually stuff it with more than it needs, it's going to have to adjust to taking in less. Within a few days, your stomach should go back to normal size and the feelings of hunger should go away. Still, help yourself not feel hungry by making sure to spread your calories as best as possible throughout the day. Don't leave yourself with too few calories for dinner. Don't dehydrate yourself by not having enough water or by having too much caffeine. This will all help to make sure that you're not left feeling empty.

Types of Food

While it's true that you can eat any kind of food as long as you count it, not all foods are going to make you *feel* the same. If you found out that a loaf of delicious, fresh-baked sourdough bread, for instance, was exactly how many calories you were allowed in a day, you might not want to limit yourself to just that sourdough bread. While this diet doesn't restrict your carbs or proteins, it's good to bear in mind that you feel best when you have both. If you just have carbs, you might feel weak and get intense cravings. If you just have chicken or meat, your body will crave the carbs. So, while it's up to you, you will likely find that something relatively balanced will be more satisfying.

Health

There's been a lot of talk about pretty much every diet that's out there in terms of whether or not it's good for you. The Atkins Diet® has been criticized up the ying-yang for supposedly contributing to cholesterol and heart disease. Most of the "detox" diets are criticized for being a shock to your body. In fact, almost every diet out there gets hammered in some way.

So what's the truth about this one? Calorie counting isn't the issue. When done in a safe way such that you're only losing one pound each week, calorie counting is usually not targeted by naysayers. But what's sure to be questioned is whether it's okay to eat hamburgers, pizza and donuts all day!

Well, duh, those foods *aren't* the healthiest out there. The point of this diet is to lower your weight. Is it encouraging you to eat unhealthy foods? No! This is for the girl that is eating that stuff *anyway*. This book just teaches you how to eat the foods you already love to eat, but in quantities that can still make you lose weight.

No one would argue against the fact that being overweight is unhealthy. Obesity is often associated with diabetes and heart disease. Losing weight can obviously help lower that risk. I know that my own cholesterol went down significantly after I lost weight, even though I wasn't (and don't) eat just lean meats and organic grass, or whatever the recommendation du jour is.

Finally, aren't there certain things everyone should have in their diet? Didn't we learn something in school about the food groups and requiring certain servings of fruit and vegetables each day? Of course. Does this diet book say *not* to eat those? *Can* you eat those with this diet? Of course. What you eat, once again, is up to you, as long as you keep track of the calories and don't exceed them.

Sometimes, as much as I want to use my last 100 calories of the day on a cookie, I use it on an apple instead. In fact, a lot of vegetables and leafy greens are extremely low in calories and can be easily accommodated in this eating plan if you so choose. In the end, you may even prefer the healthier options as they can make you feel better, and fuller.

Exercise

As long as we're on the subject of health, we might as well talk about exercise. We haven't mentioned it much thus far. After all, this is the *Lazy Girl's* weight loss method, right?

The great part about this diet is you don't need to exercise at all! That's not a joke, nor is it a lie. We've already talked about how this diet works by getting yourself to take in fewer calories than your body burns *on its own* each day. That means your body burns that amount just in carrying out its own daily processes.

When you enter your information in most of the online calorie-consumption calculators (for how many calories you need per day to lose a pound each week), it may ask you what your activity level is. As I mentioned earlier, I like to put in "sedentary" or "not active." That doesn't necessarily mean I don't have to walk in the course of my job, or lift things here and there, or that I don't occasionally actually do exercise. I do. But this way, by having the calculator count you as the lazy bum that you may or may not be, you're ensuring that this diet will be successful.

Why? For two reasons. First, let's say you put in that you are "moderately active." The calculator would then give you more calories to eat each day, because it assumes you're going to burn off those excess calories via exercise. But what if you don't exercise that day? Or what if you do exercise, but you burn fewer calories than you think you're burning? Then, those extra calories you eat will hinder (or halt) your weight loss process.

Second, by selecting "sedentary" or "inactive," you are only helping yourself lose weight. You see, if you *do* exercise at all, you're going to burn at least some calories that the calculator hadn't figured on. That means your progress in weight loss could be even *faster* than the one pound a week. It's kind of like a little bonus without having to even think about it.

But, if you really are not the typical Lazy Girl and you do actually do some exercise, if you are sure you're really burning the calories you think you are, and if you truly fit the description that the calculator gives you (i.e. "active"), then enter it that way. As with most everything in this book, it's your call.

Another important point, however, is that this eating plan's goal is to make you lose weight, i.e. fat. That means clothes will fit you a lot better, you'll feel more confident wearing that bikini again, and you'll have more energy. It doesn't, however, mean that you'll have abs of steel, rock-hard thighs, or a butt you can bounce a quarter off of. Those don't come by losing fat; they require building muscle. If that's a goal for you also, remember that this diet "only" helps you slim down, not bulk up.

However, if you do decide to build muscle, there are two important things to keep in mind. First of all, building muscle will help you burn fat more quickly and more efficiently. You might find that you lose more than a pound of fat per week when more of your fatty areas have some muscle on them. But, also remember that if you're building muscle, that old reliable bathroom scale won't give you meaningful numbers. As you may have heard, muscle weighs more than fat. So if you're gaining some muscle, the scale might actually show that you've *gained* weight, even though you're still following the plan described in this book. I, for one, prefer to do one thing at a time. I lost the fat first, and then I began building the muscle.

"Today Is Shot"

We all have days we screw up. Maybe you went out with friends and lost count of what you were eating. Maybe you found out later that something you ate had more calories than you thought. It happens.

But, don't make a bad situation worse. You can't just say, "Oh, I screwed up today. I'll go back on the diet tomorrow and it won't make a difference." Or worse yet, you can't just say, "Oh, I screwed up this afternoon. This day is shot anyway. Might as well totally indulge myself for dinner." Remember, the way this eating plan works is by counting calories. If you go over your calorie max one day by, say, 3,500 calories (a big oops), *it doesn't mean you ruined just that day*. You basically took in all the calories that you'd given up in the past seven days! It means you've put yourself back a whole week, or in terms of fat, a whole pound!

So when you screw up, don't make it any worse by screwing up more. That kind of reasoning doesn't make sense on a plan like this.

And at the same time, don't beat yourself up. We all have off days, but the key is to have them as seldom as possible.

The Weigh-In

Of course the key to this eating plan is losing fat. The best way to see a difference is by using that reflective glass in the bathroom – your mirror. But just checking yourself out is not a very accurate way to measure weight loss. Besides, you might not notice the difference right away.

So the first thing you need to do is go buy a scale, preferably a digital one. Now there's no need to go buy the most expensive one (unless you want to), but don't go for the cheapest one either. Since we're talking about losing one pound a week, you want a scale that's very accurate.

Also, don't weigh yourself every day. It'll wreak havoc on your mind. Yes, technically you should be losing 1/7 of a pound each day or 0.14 pounds, but even if you have a scale that is that exact, the weight loss won't necessarily show up that way. It depends on how much water you've had, whether you've used the toilet, if it's that time of the month, and other factors.

So the best way to track your weight changes is to weigh yourself at the same time every week. You should do it without clothes, after you've done your business, before you've had anything to eat or drink, and preferably in the morning. You'd be surprised how much more you weigh in the afternoon and evening.

Tracking Calories

This is the only part that requires Lazy Girls to do a little work. But no, it doesn't involve exercise. It doesn't involve chopping something, preparing anything, or buying something weird at the grocery store.

Unless you have a calculator in your head, for this eating program to work, you're going to need to track your calories. I usually just jot it down on a piece of paper (like Britney did) as soon as I eat something (or right after, when none of my friends are watching.)

You want to be as accurate as possible. So don't round or estimate, unless it's absolutely necessary. Miscalculations add up, and they could leave you disappointed at the end of a couple of weeks.

You can keep a running total, as such:

Friday, 1/10/2013

Bagel	330
With tablespoon of cream cheese	60
Half of a donut	220
Chicken parmesan sandwich	670
Total so far today:	1,280

Or you can keep track of what you have left, as such:

Friday, 1/10/2013
      Bagel   330
      With tablespoon of cream cheese   60
      Half of a donut   220
      Chicken parmesan sandwich   670

            Remaining today: $1300 - 1280 = 20$

Either way, whichever works for you. But you must count everything. That little red-and-white peppermint candy you took after lunch counts. (Hard to find in the nutritional information sources, but it's about 30 calories.) So do the ketchup packet you used for your fries, the parmesan cheese you sprinkled on your rigatoni, and the cinnamon stick that came in your milkshake.

Eating Times

You've no doubt heard the idea that you should never eat after a certain time at night or you'll gain (or not lose) weight. However, I've read that this is just a myth, and that if you take in less than you burn, you'll still lose weight, no matter what time of day it is. So I wouldn't worry about this one. I could, however, see how it's better to not eat *right* before you go to sleep because you don't burn as many calories asleep as you do awake, but I've noticed that the program still works even if I do.

A Thinner Future

From this point on, you're on your own, my Lazy Girl child. I've given you the resources and shown you how you can get rid of your extra load in the easiest possible way, and still enjoy eating. Set a goal weight and a goal date. You might want to work in small steps, like 5 or 10 pounds at a time and then reassess once you get there. Refer back to this book when necessary to remind yourself of the basics and the possibilities.

When you get to your final goal weight, don't make the too common mistake of gaining it all back. Go back to your old friend, the online calorie-consumption calculator, and see how much you can eat to *maintain* your weight. (It will be a much higher number.) Try your best to keep your consumption under that number. If you go up a little, you'll be okay. After all, now you know how to lose it the Lazy Girl's way.

Good luck, and remember, losing weight doesn't have to be brutal misery, just basic math.

Appendix A:
Online Calorie-Consumption Calculators

A Few Reliable Calorie-Consumption Calculators
http://www.mayoclinic.com/health/calorie-calculator/NU00598
http://www.freedieting.com/tools/calorie_calculator.htm
http://calorieneedscalculator.com/
http://www.healthyweightforum.org/eng/calculators/calories-required/
http://www.caloriesperhour.com/
http://www.hpathy.com/healthtools/calories-need.asp

Appendix B:
Online Nutritional Information Sources (N.I.S.)

www.calorielab.com
www.calorieking.com
www.caloriescount.com
www.caloriecountercharts.com
www.nutritiondata.com
www.nal.usda.gov/fnic/foodcomp/search
www.calorie-charts.net

Appendix C: Calorie Tracker Sheet

Week #	Sunday		Monday		Tuesday		Wednesday		Thursday		Friday		Saturday	
/ / through / /	Item	Cal.	Item	Cal.	Item	Cal.	Item	Cal.	Item	Cal.	Item	Cal.	Item	Cal.
Begin. Wt.:														
Notes:														